Ketogenic Diet Recipe

TABLE OF CONTENTS

/PAGE/	/RECIPE NAME/	/NOTES/

TABLE OF CONTENTS

/PAGE/	/RECIPE NAME/	/NOTES/

TABLE OF CONTENTS

/PAGE/	/RECIPE NAME/	/NOTES/

Recipe

Ingredient	Amount

Direction

Nutrition

Serving Size	Carb	Pro	Fat	Calories

Note

Recipe

Ingredient	Amount

Direction

Nutrition

Serving Size	Carb	Pro	Fat	Calories

Note

Recipe

Ingredient	Amount

Direction

Nutrition

Serving Size	Carb	Pro	Fat	Calories

Note

Recipe

Ingredient	Amount

Direction

Nutrition

Serving Size	Carb	Pro	Fat	Calories

Note

Recipe

Ingredient	Amount

Direction

Nutrition

Serving Size	Carb	Pro	Fat	Calories

Note

Recipe

Ingredient	Amount

Direction

Nutrition

Serving Size	Carb	Pro	Fat	Calories

Note

Recipe

Ingredient	Amount

Direction

Nutrition

Serving Size	Carb	Pro	Fat	Calories

Note

Recipe

Ingredient	Amount

Direction

Nutrition

Serving Size	Carb	Pro	Fat	Calories

Note

Recipe

Ingredient	Amount

Direction

Nutrition

Serving Size	Carb	Pro	Fat	Calories

Note

Recipe

Ingredient	Amount

Direction

Nutrition

Serving Size	Carb	Pro	Fat	Calories

Note

Recipe

Ingredient	Amount

Direction

Nutrition

Serving Size	Carb	Pro	Fat	Calories

Note

Recipe

Ingredient	Amount

Direction

Nutrition

Serving Size	Carb	Pro	Fat	Calories

Note

Recipe

Ingredient	Amount

Direction

Nutrition

Serving Size	Carb	Pro	Fat	Calories

Note

Recipe

Ingredient	Amount

Direction

Nutrition

Serving Size	Carb	Pro	Fat	Calories

Note

Recipe

Ingredient	Amount

Direction

Nutrition

Serving Size	Carb	Pro	Fat	Calories

Note

Recipe

Ingredient	Amount

Direction

Nutrition

Serving Size	Carb	Pro	Fat	Calories

Note

Recipe

Ingredient	Amount

Direction

Nutrition

Serving Size	Carb	Pro	Fat	Calories

Note

Recipe

Ingredient	Amount

Direction

Nutrition

Serving Size	Carb	Pro	Fat	Calories

Note

Recipe

Ingredient	Amount

Direction

Nutrition

Serving Size	Carb	Pro	Fat	Calories

Note

Recipe

Ingredient	Amount

Direction

Nutrition

Serving Size	Carb	Pro	Fat	Calories

Note

Recipe

Ingredient	Amount

Direction

Nutrition

Serving Size	Carb	Pro	Fat	Calories

Note

Recipe

Ingredient	Amount

Direction

Nutrition

Serving Size	Carb	Pro	Fat	Calories

Note

Recipe

Ingredient	Amount

Direction

Nutrition

Serving Size	Carb	Pro	Fat	Calories

Note

Recipe

Ingredient	Amount

Direction

Nutrition

Serving Size	Carb	Pro	Fat	Calories

Note

Recipe

Ingredient	Amount

Direction

Nutrition

Serving Size	Carb	Pro	Fat	Calories

Note

Recipe

Ingredient	Amount

Direction

Nutrition

Serving Size	Carb	Pro	Fat	Calories

Note

Recipe

Ingredient	Amount

Direction

Nutrition

Serving Size	Carb	Pro	Fat	Calories

Note

Recipe

Ingredient	Amount

Direction

Nutrition

Serving Size	Carb	Pro	Fat	Calories

Note

Recipe

Ingredient	Amount

Direction

Nutrition

Serving Size	Carb	Pro	Fat	Calories

Note

Recipe

Ingredient	Amount

Direction

Nutrition

Serving Size	Carb	Pro	Fat	Calories

Note

Recipe

Ingredient	Amount

Direction

Nutrition

Serving Size	Carb	Pro	Fat	Calories

Note

Recipe

Ingredient	Amount

Direction

Nutrition

Serving Size	Carb	Pro	Fat	Calories

Note

Recipe

Ingredient	Amount

Direction

Nutrition

Serving Size	Carb	Pro	Fat	Calories

Note

Recipe

Ingredient	Amount

Direction

Nutrition

Serving Size	Carb	Pro	Fat	Calories

Note

Recipe

Ingredient	Amount

Direction

Nutrition

Serving Size	Carb	Pro	Fat	Calories

Note

Recipe

Ingredient	Amount

Direction

Nutrition

Serving Size	Carb	Pro	Fat	Calories

Note

Recipe

Ingredient	Amount

Direction

Nutrition

Serving Size	Carb	Pro	Fat	Calories

Note

Recipe

Ingredient	Amount

Direction

Nutrition

Serving Size	Carb	Pro	Fat	Calories

Note

Recipe

Ingredient	Amount

Direction

Nutrition

Serving Size	Carb	Pro	Fat	Calories

Note

Recipe

Ingredient	Amount

Direction

Nutrition

Serving Size	Carb	Pro	Fat	Calories

Note

Recipe

Ingredient	Amount

Direction

Nutrition

Serving Size	Carb	Pro	Fat	Calories

Note

Recipe

Ingredient	Amount

Direction

Nutrition

Serving Size	Carb	Pro	Fat	Calories

Note

Recipe

Ingredient	Amount

Direction

Nutrition

Serving Size	Carb	Pro	Fat	Calories

Note

Recipe

Ingredient	Amount

Direction

Nutrition

Serving Size	Carb	Pro	Fat	Calories

Note

Recipe

Ingredient	Amount

Direction

Nutrition

Serving Size	Carb	Pro	Fat	Calories

Note

Recipe

Ingredient	Amount

Direction

Nutrition

Serving Size	Carb	Pro	Fat	Calories

Note

Recipe

Ingredient	Amount

Direction

Nutrition

Serving Size	Carb	Pro	Fat	Calories

Note

Recipe

Ingredient	Amount

Direction

Nutrition

Serving Size	Carb	Pro	Fat	Calories

Note

Recipe

Ingredient	Amount

Direction

Nutrition

Serving Size	Carb	Pro	Fat	Calories

Note

Recipe

Ingredient	Amount

Direction

Nutrition

Serving Size	Carb	Pro	Fat	Calories

Note

Recipe

Ingredient	Amount

Direction

Nutrition

Serving Size	Carb	Pro	Fat	Calories

Note

Recipe

Ingredient	Amount

Direction

Nutrition

Serving Size	Carb	Pro	Fat	Calories

Note

Recipe

Ingredient	Amount

Direction

Nutrition

Serving Size	Carb	Pro	Fat	Calories

Note

Recipe

Ingredient	Amount

Direction

Nutrition

Serving Size	Carb	Pro	Fat	Calories

Note

Recipe

Ingredient	Amount

Direction

Nutrition

Serving Size	Carb	Pro	Fat	Calories

Note

Recipe

Ingredient	Amount

Direction

Nutrition

Serving Size	Carb	Pro	Fat	Calories

Note

Recipe

Ingredient	Amount

Direction

Nutrition

Serving Size	Carb	Pro	Fat	Calories

Note

Recipe

Ingredient	Amount

Direction

Nutrition

Serving Size	Carb	Pro	Fat	Calories

Note

Recipe

Ingredient	Amount

Direction

Nutrition

Serving Size	Carb	Pro	Fat	Calories

Note

Recipe

Ingredient	Amount

Direction

Nutrition

Serving Size	Carb	Pro	Fat	Calories

Note

Recipe

Ingredient	Amount

Direction

Nutrition

Serving Size	Carb	Pro	Fat	Calories

Note

Recipe

Ingredient	Amount

Direction

Nutrition

Serving Size	Carb	Pro	Fat	Calories

Note

Recipe

Ingredient	Amount

Direction

Nutrition

Serving Size	Carb	Pro	Fat	Calories

Note

Recipe

Ingredient	Amount

Direction

Nutrition

Serving Size	Carb	Pro	Fat	Calories

Note

Recipe

Ingredient	Amount

Direction

Nutrition

Serving Size	Carb	Pro	Fat	Calories

Note

Recipe

Ingredient	Amount

Direction

Nutrition

Serving Size	Carb	Pro	Fat	Calories

Note

Recipe

Ingredient	Amount

Direction

Nutrition

Serving Size	Carb	Pro	Fat	Calories

Note

Recipe

Ingredient	Amount

Direction

Nutrition

Serving Size	Carb	Pro	Fat	Calories

Note

Recipe

Ingredient	Amount

Direction

Nutrition

Serving Size	Carb	Pro	Fat	Calories

Note

Recipe

Ingredient	Amount

Direction

Nutrition

Serving Size	Carb	Pro	Fat	Calories

Note

Recipe

Ingredient	Amount

Direction

Nutrition

Serving Size	Carb	Pro	Fat	Calories

Note

Recipe

Ingredient	Amount

Direction

Nutrition

Serving Size	Carb	Pro	Fat	Calories

Note

Recipe

Ingredient	Amount

Direction

Nutrition

Serving Size	Carb	Pro	Fat	Calories

Note

Recipe

Ingredient	Amount

Direction

Nutrition

Serving Size	Carb	Pro	Fat	Calories

Note

Recipe

Ingredient	Amount

Direction

Nutrition

Serving Size	Carb	Pro	Fat	Calories

Note

Recipe

Ingredient	Amount

Direction

Nutrition

Serving Size	Carb	Pro	Fat	Calories

Note

Recipe

Ingredient	Amount

Direction

Nutrition

Serving Size	Carb	Pro	Fat	Calories

Note

Recipe

Ingredient	Amount

Direction

Nutrition

Serving Size	Carb	Pro	Fat	Calories

Note

Recipe

Ingredient	Amount

Direction

Nutrition

Serving Size	Carb	Pro	Fat	Calories

Note

Recipe

Ingredient	Amount

Direction

Nutrition

Serving Size	Carb	Pro	Fat	Calories

Note

Recipe

Ingredient	Amount

Direction

Nutrition

Serving Size	Carb	Pro	Fat	Calories

Note

Recipe

Ingredient	Amount

Direction

Nutrition

Serving Size	Carb	Pro	Fat	Calories

Note

Recipe

Ingredient	Amount

Direction

Nutrition

Serving Size	Carb	Pro	Fat	Calories

Note

Recipe

Ingredient	Amount

Direction

Nutrition

Serving Size	Carb	Pro	Fat	Calories

Note

Recipe

Ingredient	Amount

Direction

Nutrition

Serving Size	Carb	Pro	Fat	Calories

Note

Recipe

Ingredient	Amount

Direction

Nutrition

Serving Size	Carb	Pro	Fat	Calories

Note

Recipe

Ingredient	Amount

Direction

Nutrition

Serving Size	Carb	Pro	Fat	Calories

Note

Recipe

Ingredient	Amount

Direction

Nutrition

Serving Size	Carb	Pro	Fat	Calories

Note

Recipe

Ingredient	Amount

Direction

Nutrition

Serving Size	Carb	Pro	Fat	Calories

Note

Recipe

Ingredient	Amount

Direction

Nutrition

Serving Size	Carb	Pro	Fat	Calories

Note

Recipe

Ingredient	Amount

Direction

Nutrition

Serving Size	Carb	Pro	Fat	Calories

Note

Recipe

Ingredient	Amount

Direction

Nutrition

Serving Size	Carb	Pro	Fat	Calories

Note

Recipe

Ingredient	Amount

Direction

Nutrition

Serving Size	Carb	Pro	Fat	Calories

Note

Recipe

Ingredient	Amount

Direction

Nutrition

Serving Size	Carb	Pro	Fat	Calories

Note

Recipe

Ingredient	Amount

Direction

Nutrition

Serving Size	Carb	Pro	Fat	Calories

Note

Recipe

Ingredient	Amount

Direction

Nutrition

Serving Size	Carb	Pro	Fat	Calories

Note

Recipe

Ingredient	Amount

Direction

Nutrition

Serving Size	Carb	Pro	Fat	Calories

Note

Recipe

Ingredient	Amount

Direction

Nutrition

Serving Size	Carb	Pro	Fat	Calories

Note

Recipe

Ingredient	Amount

Direction

Nutrition

Serving Size	Carb	Pro	Fat	Calories

Note

Recipe

Ingredient	Amount

Direction

Nutrition

Serving Size	Carb	Pro	Fat	Calories

Note

Recipe

Ingredient	Amount

Direction

Nutrition

Serving Size	Carb	Pro	Fat	Calories

Note

Recipe

Ingredient	Amount

Direction

Nutrition

Serving Size	Carb	Pro	Fat	Calories

Note

Recipe

Ingredient	Amount

Direction

Nutrition

Serving Size	Carb	Pro	Fat	Calories

Note

Recipe

Ingredient	Amount

Direction

Nutrition

Serving Size	Carb	Pro	Fat	Calories

Note

Recipe

Ingredient	Amount

Direction

Nutrition

Serving Size	Carb	Pro	Fat	Calories

Note

Recipe

Ingredient	Amount

Direction

Nutrition

Serving Size	Carb	Pro	Fat	Calories

Note

Recipe

Ingredient	Amount

Direction

Nutrition

Serving Size	Carb	Pro	Fat	Calories

Note

Recipe

Ingredient	Amount

Direction

Nutrition

Serving Size	Carb	Pro	Fat	Calories

Note

Recipe

Ingredient	Amount

Direction

Nutrition

Serving Size	Carb	Pro	Fat	Calories

Note

Recipe

Ingredient	Amount

Direction

Nutrition

Serving Size	Carb	Pro	Fat	Calories

Note

Recipe

Ingredient	Amount

Direction

Nutrition

Serving Size	Carb	Pro	Fat	Calories

Note

Recipe

Ingredient	Amount

Direction

Nutrition

Serving Size	Carb	Pro	Fat	Calories

Note

Recipe

Ingredient	Amount

Direction

Nutrition

Serving Size	Carb	Pro	Fat	Calories

Note

Recipe

Ingredient	Amount

Direction

Nutrition

Serving Size	Carb	Pro	Fat	Calories

Note

Recipe

Ingredient	Amount

Direction

Nutrition

Serving Size	Carb	Pro	Fat	Calories

Note

Recipe

Ingredient	Amount

Direction

Nutrition

Serving Size	Carb	Pro	Fat	Calories

Note

Recipe

Ingredient	Amount

Direction

Nutrition

Serving Size	Carb	Pro	Fat	Calories

Note

Recipe

Ingredient	Amount

Direction

Nutrition

Serving Size	Carb	Pro	Fat	Calories

Note

Recipe

Ingredient	Amount

Direction

Nutrition

Serving Size	Carb	Pro	Fat	Calories

Note

Recipe

Ingredient	Amount

Direction

Nutrition

Serving Size	Carb	Pro	Fat	Calories

Note

Recipe

Ingredient	Amount

Direction

Nutrition

Serving Size	Carb	Pro	Fat	Calories

Note

Recipe

Ingredient	Amount

Direction

Nutrition

Serving Size	Carb	Pro	Fat	Calories

Note

Recipe

Ingredient	Amount

Direction

Nutrition

Serving Size	Carb	Pro	Fat	Calories

Note

Recipe

Ingredient	Amount

Direction

Nutrition

Serving Size	Carb	Pro	Fat	Calories

Note

Recipe

Ingredient	Amount

Direction

Nutrition

Serving Size	Carb	Pro	Fat	Calories

Note

Recipe

Ingredient	Amount

Direction

Nutrition

Serving Size	Carb	Pro	Fat	Calories

Note

Recipe

Ingredient	Amount

Direction

Nutrition

Serving Size	Carb	Pro	Fat	Calories

Note

Recipe

Ingredient	Amount

Direction

Nutrition

Serving Size	Carb	Pro	Fat	Calories

Note

Recipe

Ingredient	Amount

Direction

Nutrition

Serving Size	Carb	Pro	Fat	Calories

Note

Recipe

Ingredient	Amount

Direction

Nutrition

Serving Size	Carb	Pro	Fat	Calories

Note

Recipe

Ingredient	Amount

Direction

Nutrition

Serving Size	Carb	Pro	Fat	Calories

Note

Recipe

Ingredient	Amount

Direction

Nutrition

Serving Size	Carb	Pro	Fat	Calories

Note

Recipe

Ingredient	Amount

Direction

Nutrition

Serving Size	Carb	Pro	Fat	Calories

Note

Recipe

Ingredient	Amount

Direction

Nutrition

Serving Size	Carb	Pro	Fat	Calories

Note

Recipe

Ingredient	Amount

Direction

Nutrition

Serving Size	Carb	Pro	Fat	Calories

Note

Recipe

Ingredient	Amount

Direction

Nutrition

Serving Size	Carb	Pro	Fat	Calories

Note

Recipe

Ingredient	Amount

Direction

Nutrition

Serving Size	Carb	Pro	Fat	Calories

Note

Recipe

Ingredient	Amount

Direction

Nutrition

Serving Size	Carb	Pro	Fat	Calories

Note

Recipe

Ingredient	Amount

Direction

Nutrition

Serving Size	Carb	Pro	Fat	Calories

Note

Recipe

Ingredient	Amount

Direction

Nutrition

Serving Size	Carb	Pro	Fat	Calories

Note

Recipe

Ingredient	Amount

Direction

Nutrition

Serving Size	Carb	Pro	Fat	Calories

Note

Recipe

Ingredient	Amount

Direction

Nutrition

Serving Size	Carb	Pro	Fat	Calories

Note

Recipe

Ingredient	Amount

Direction

Nutrition

Serving Size	Carb	Pro	Fat	Calories

Note

Recipe

Ingredient	Amount

Direction

Nutrition

Serving Size	Carb	Pro	Fat	Calories

Note

Recipe

Ingredient	Amount

Direction

Nutrition

Serving Size	Carb	Pro	Fat	Calories

Note

Recipe

Ingredient	Amount

Direction

Nutrition

Serving Size	Carb	Pro	Fat	Calories

Note

Recipe

Ingredient	Amount

Direction

Nutrition

Serving Size	Carb	Pro	Fat	Calories

Note

Recipe

Ingredient	Amount

Direction

Nutrition

Serving Size	Carb	Pro	Fat	Calories

Note

Recipe

Ingredient	Amount

Direction

Nutrition

Serving Size	Carb	Pro	Fat	Calories

Note

Recipe

Ingredient	Amount

Direction

Nutrition

Serving Size	Carb	Pro	Fat	Calories

Note